WHITE EFFECT

The white coat effect on the doctor-patient relationship

WHITE EFFECT

The white coat effect on the doctor-patient relationship

Edited by
Gianna Pamich

Foreword
Gerhard Konrad Seeberger

edra

Book Publishing Manager: Arianna Ribichesu

Book Project Manager: Giulia Barollo

Cover: Ursula Giusti

ISBN: 978-88-214-5700-5
eISBN: 978-88-214-5701-2

Edra S.p.A.
Via G. Spadolini 7
20141 Milano
Tel. 02 881841
www.edizioniedra.it

Printed in Italy, May 2022 by "LegoDigit" Srl., Lavis (TN)

(*) Edra S.p.A. is part of LSWR GROUP

FOREWORD

WHITE COAT AND SCIENCE, INSEPARABLE COMPANIONS

The white coat has its roots in the Arabic word 'qamiç', meaning a tunic, a long, white linen underrobe worn by priests during the celebration of divine offices, but also in the Greek word 'kámasos', a square-shaped, sleeveless garment made of cotton, linen, or silk.

The ancient Romans used it as an undergarment and adopted the Hellenic name. The first ones were beige, then they took on various colors depending on the activity of professionals and artists. However, the first person to wear a white coat was not a doctor.

Historical examples of medical practice can be found in India with Ayurveda, in Saudi Arabia with the practice of prophetic medicine, in Greece with the Hippocratic Yunānī as well as in the Roman and Byzantine Empires. However, the oldest medical profession is still dentistry, dating back to 7000 BC, the time of the Indus Valley Civilization. No ancient healer was distinguished by his white coats.

About 2500 years ago modern medicine split from ancient medicine, the one linked to the supernatural, to philosophical and theurgic practices and the belief that diseases were caused by evil demons or were the consequence of offences against the gods. Hippocrates of Kos invented the medical record, theorized the need to observe the patient considering his 'symptoms' and the concepts of 'diagnosis' and 'prognosis'.

The doctor finally became a pragmatic observer who based his diagnosis on scientific criteria, a man who helped patients following the *primum nihil nocere* principle and did not keep his knowledge to himself, but taught it to his disciples, treating them as brothers and sisters.

Medicine became transparent and ethical. The dark medieval times were lit up by the *Canon of Medicine*. Introduced at the beginning of the second millennium by Ibn Sīnā, aka Abū ʿAlī al-Ḥusayn ibn ʿAbd Allāh ibn Sīnā, known in the West as Avicenna, the *Canon* was to become the most widely followed manual of medicine in Europe until the eighteenth century.

In 1723 Pierre Fauchard, the father of modern dentistry, published the historic book *The Surgical Dentist or Treatise on the Teeth*. The time was ripe to represent all medicine with the white colour, which expressed purity, hope, and transformation.

The white coat came about in laboratories and, before becoming the symbol of modern medicine at the end of the nineteenth century, became the symbol of a science that put an end to the dark times of the Middle Ages and to the heavy, protective scrub made of leather and the black doctor scrub.

At that time the world saw the first commercial automobile powered by an internal combustion engine, designed by Karl Friedrich Benz, as well as the production of the electric light bulb by Thomas Edison and Alessandro Cruto, and the discovery of X-rays by Wilhelm Conrad Röntgen on November 8, 1895.

It was right Röntgen, Nobel prize for physics, who combined the white lab coat with the doctor scrub when he was awarded an honorary degree in medicine by the University of Würzburg, Germany.

Röntgen paved the way for diagnostic imaging, giving physicians the opportunity to learn more about the human body; so did Louis Pasteur, Joseph Lister and Robert Koch with regard to the understanding of infectious diseases and prevention, particularly during surgeries.

The white coat was such also for the low cost of the fabric, to allow a rapid detection of its contamination and better withstand the high temperatures of the washing and sterilization process. In addition to having become a symbol of purity for medicine and the garment itself, it is regarded a guarantee for the operator's and patient's safety.

The physician in a white coat gains credibility among patients; he is attributed more authority, compassion, credibility, and experience. A very recent survey of 522 patients found that physicians in informal attire are considered less professional and experienced than those wearing white coats.

In the late twentieth century, except for periods of emergency due to wars or natural disasters, doctors used the white coat not so much for protection as for identification purposes. Identifying a white coat quickly meant life and survival. But those who wore that color were not always physicians.

In hospitals and large healthcare units, nurses, clinic managers, epidemiologists, pharmacists, and many others also wore white clothes. The white coat needed to be coloured, not only in operating rooms where green (the colour still preferred by surgeons) was adopted to facilitate the operator's visual concentration, and not to confuse the patient.

Thus, the white coat became an 'informer' because of its colour and style. The patient had the right to know which health worker took care of him, so the white colour influenced the individual health outcome. In times of unrestrained information, it has also become a messenger for advertising space, turning the wearer into a living billboard column.

The colour had also to serve a psychological function. To reduce patients' anxiety, pediatricians and psychologists have abandoned the white coat and have long been presenting themselves in multicoloured garments with designs known to the youngest patients, or in informal attire: this is the case of the psychologist, who does not necessarily need to have physical contact with the patient.

However, the colour does not solve a fundamental aspect of the doctor scrub: its cleanliness. Studies have shown that the white coat is almost as much a vehicle to carry diseases as money and other objects contaminated by myriad of hands, more or less clean. A study showed that it was washed by hospital staff on average every 12 days and because of this, it was soon replaced with disposable garments.

This expedient proved indispensable in the early days of the Covid-19 outbreak but involves a super-production of waste. The threat to the environment urged to find other solutions, which science promptly provided. Photodynamic layers of cross-linked polymers and photosensitive materials applied to doctors' white coats can guarantee almost total inactivation of bacteria and viruses for 4 weeks. And science can make colours useful again even in the worst emergencies.

The photosensitive material is in rose bengal, a bluish-red color which alone inactivates 99.97% of staphylococcus aureus on wool-acrylic blended fabrics when exposed to visible light, while the addition of cationic colours such as yellow, blue, and red, decreases this value to 99.30%.

If we want to describe the status quo of the white coat and at the same time look to its future, we could say that the white coat and science are and will remain inseparable companions. Whoever wears it should never betray it, as the white coat never betrays the healthcare provider.

The confidence in the wearer's competence and experience, the hope of receiving help from those who operate in transparency on the basis of knowledge and know-how, purity expressed in the colour and compassion of the medical figure make those who wear it and the 'white' coat itself timeless stars.

Gerhard Konrad Seeberger
Past President FDI World Dental Federation
Immediate Past President Academy of Dentistry International

PREFACE

If an investigation was made of the story, facts, psychological aspects, colours, shape, times of use, regulations on the fabric etc. among 'insiders', few would be able to answer, as they would refer to personal habits or generalised customs.

And yet, behind the white coat or mismatched outfit–an item of clothing which, according to an authoritative insider, 'is given the same attention as a shoelace'–rises a wide range of reflections, some of which could even take us far; to various surprises, in any case.

We will discover them a bit at a time through the various chapters of this text. Let us say right away that we will disregard the countless types of scrubs currently used in various trades and/or professions. We will focus on the role played by the white coat in the doctor-patient relationship and, in more detail, in the odontologist-patient relationship.

Gianna Pamich

AKNOWLEDGEMENTS

For the passion and relish shown in their work, I would like to thank:

Stefano Almini

Fausto Assandri

Massimo Boccaletti

Silvana Graziana Ceresa

Francesco Colosimo

Carlo Guastamacchia

Elena Pozzani

Maria Sofia Rini

Index

Chapter 1

GAMES OF THE UNCONSCIOUS

'It is a garment with a great symbolic importance'. This is the definition that Silvana Graziella Ceresa, a psychotherapist and jungian analyst, gives when she is asked to label the white coat from a psychological point of view. The white coat is a garment which, after all, is also worn by pharmacists, nurses, laboratory technicians, biologists and chemists and all of them operate in healthcare work environments with important hygienic requirements, where the white coat has a symbolic charge.

However, painters and restorers too wear it to distinguish themselves professionally and better protect themselves from stains, as also do operators in any butcher's shop.

But what's the relation between the 'white coats'–as physicians are commonly called–and others, who are also white-clad? With a broader look, we learn from psychology that mental processes derive from received perceptions; not only from material and immediately tangible elements like fabric and colour, but also from symbolic meanings which, totally unconsciously, are attributed to received stimuli.

There is a particular relationship between attire and psyche; it is an unconscious allurement deriving from use made of clothes, which researchers call "priming effect".

If you think carefully about it–she continues–choosing a garment often requires careful attention to the place where it is worn and to the people you encounter, because attire is perceived by others in a specific way. Everyone reacts to the received perception, to the point of conditioning his own behavior and thoughts, which results in unconscious attitude and even personal performance changes.

From perception to fruition. A garment is like a second skin: if we feel at ease in that 'coating', we become more social and assume a more confident behavior. Conversely, if we feel ill at ease in it, the whole pattern of relations with ourselves and others is affected. We can rightly say, therefore, that individual performances are influenced by our clothes. Hence the importance of wearing clothes symbolising the desired effect: a creative/professional, chaste/seducing, serious/amusing one.

According to the psychologist's revelations, the uniforms, and the formal clothes in general, have an important impact on people's behavior, as they become primarily an official symbol of knowledge and know-how. A tidy white coat or a crumpled one, after a long and tiring use (two extremes of the evaluation of excellence) symbolise professional efficiency.

Each individual can be defined through a personal identity linked to the role and aspects that make him different from others, and through a social identity related to the group he belongs to: social characterisations, in fact, make the status of the person observed immediately perceivable to the observer's mind. Attire provides the reference in a directly accessible way.

Social identity distinguishes people's behavior. The uniform or another shared, distinguishing attire become a distinctive, elitist sign. Identification is suggested by the clothes which express the role, functions and degree through compliance with often unspecified rules which are yet essential for the group. Any institution is regulated by stated, shared norms, but is governed, even controlled, by undeclared, unspecified yet vital rules.

Many studies have been conducted on what has been called 'embodied cognition', which directly relates body and mind. The 'embodied mind' thesis, which great psychoanalyst Francisco Varela enunciated in 1987, meant having a body with sensorimotor skills embodied in a complex psychological, biological, cultural context in which the group a person belongs to plays a significant role.

Other studies carried out by Adams and Galinsky in 2012 examine the concept of 'enclothed cognition' which is related to two elements: the symbolical meaning of a garment and the way it is worn, that is, its effect on the mental, personal and/or collective process. As it turned out, expectations of a person are closely linked to the image he places on himself through his behavior, his clothes, and the way he wears them. What re-emerges is the concept of the person who is believed to know and know how to do.

It is an unconscious game. It is assumed that he knows what the interlocutor wants to know, gaining trust from the start, and to know how to do according to the clothes he wears. According to a survey published by the American Journal of Medicine in 2005, patients are believed to place more trust in a doctor in a scrub (better if traditionally white) than in another doctor wearing a scrub with a different style or even none.

The research carried out in a waiting room of an American clinic consisted in a written questionnaire with enclosed pictures of physicians in 4 different outfits. Patients had to indicate which doctor they preferred and to whom they would be more willing to reveal their own problems.

A good 76.3% of the interviewees admitted they would prefer a doctor 'in professional attire' (that is, in white coat). The percentage was even higher if attire regarded a woman doctor.

We learn from Adn Kronos that also according to the Department of Epidemiology of the University Hospital of Zurich, the colour influences the success of a treatment: a study confirms that 'patients appear to be more trusting if a doctor wears a white coat' and makes it clear that the goal 'is not to find out what is pleasant to the patients' eyes, but rather their mostly unconscious reaction to the appearance of doctors.'

The answers to questions such as which clothes inspire more trust, in which outfit physicians appear more helpful and approachable, and if it is true that patients attribute professional skills to a certain type of attire, lead all and inevitably to the white coat, as Head of Department Hugo Sax confirms. According to this investigation, in which 834 patients were involved, a third of the interviewees believe that the doctor's look is very important, while about 25% believe that attire also influences the opinion on treatment.

Later on, from the observations made by a well-known master of dentistry in respect of the 'appropriate' look of a professional, we will see that practice confirms the statistical results. However, a first, nearly conclusive reflection arises spontaneously even if we are at the beginning of this treatise: probably there is 'nothing new under the sun'. Even Hippocrates Koo, nearly 2500 years ago, recommended wearing, if not white, at least appropriate clothes. A therapist and psychologist ahead of his time, he had already noticed that 'these details have a positive impact on patients.'

Chapter 2

REMBRANDT'S HAT

It is difficult to find a painting as well-known as *The anatomy lesson of Dr. Tulp* by Rembrandt Harmenszoon van Rijn, a painter from Leiden, Netherlands, better known as Rembrandt. Considered a leading exponent of European art and the main protagonist of the 'Dutch Golden Age', this prolific artist is believed to be the author of about 300 works, among which about 100 self-portraits.

The aforesaid painting, which Rembrandt did in 1636 at the age of 26, is not only known for being one of his first masterpieces; it is also familiar in the healthcare field for a somewhat trivial reason.

Let us see, therefore, why the famous *Lesson* showing Dr. Tulp, City Anatomist of Amsterdam, explaining the physiology of the arm to some doctors, could hold a prominent position in the multifaceted role played by the white coat in the doctor-patient relationship.

If death, legally speaking, is the event that turns a person, a rights holder into a 'thing', then Aris Kindt too (also known as Adriaan Adriaanszoon), convicted of robbery, is here turned, after being hanged, into an object–in this case, an object particularly worthy of study, at least judging from the attention the portrayed medical 'students' pay to the dissection, a procedure which, according to reports, took place once a year, was open to the public and performed on the corpse of an executed person.

As it is impossible to find any trace of white coats in a 1632 painting albeit showing a few physicians and an academic surgeon teaching his lesson, it is necessary to wait about two and a half centuries (1889) to find the first painting representing a white coat. It is called *The Agnew Clinic*. A work by the American artist Thomas Eakins, it depicts an operation carried out by white-clad surgeons, the only difference being that they intervene on a sick person and not on the body of an executed man. History, however, runs fast.

About fifteen years earlier (1875), in another painting entitled *The Gross Clinic*, Eakins had portrayed some surgeons performing an operation but wearing no scrub, as was customary then. Over everyone dominates Samuel Gross, an authoritative professor who explains to the students of the Jefferson Medical College the various steps of the surgery.

As a doctor scrub he wears an elegant black garment–black being the traditional color of the medical profession (ed.)–which would soon give a way to a new, completely different, predominantly white professional device, still in use today.

Coming back to Dr. Nicolaes Tulp and his lecture, we see that here too the progenitor of today's white coat is represented by the elegant black garment worn by the City Anatomist. It is an obvious status symbol which, though not appearing as such in the eyes of the 'patient' (who has become a corpse, therefore a 'thing'), is viewed as such by the society of that time and by the same doctors/students eagerly staring at 'the thing' to get its secrets.

At a closer look, the painting shows even two status symbols, as is often the case in our age as well. In addition to Tulp's refined black robe (the first status symbol), it is no mere coincidence that Rembrandt portrayed all his pupils bareheaded, while only the 'protophysicist' (to quote a term used by Manzoni) wears a hat as a further sign of distinction (second status symbol).

That wide-brimmed hat may appear as a sort of forerunner symbol of the modern white coat that sometimes, at least judging from some images of the past (but also from the testimony of some 'not-so-young' clinicians), became 'longer' if the wearer held a higher position in the medical hierarchy.

The famous dissection was not the only one represented by Rembrandt in his fabulous career, because about twenty years later (1656) the great master gave birth to a similar masterpiece to be exhibited in the Anatomical Room of Amsterdam together with the previous one.

Entitled *The lesson of Dr. Deijman*, Tulp's successor as City Anatomist, it was damaged by fire in 1723, so only the central part has remained, enlivened by two figures: one on the left, the other, half-hidden behind the head of the corpse, portrayed with the bust erect.

That fire was a double, real shame. In fact, following the interpretation given to Tulp's attire, it would have been useful, to confirm the hypothesis of the double status symbol, to ascertain which attire was attributed by Rembrandt to Dr. Dejiman. But because of the fire, that hypothesis, albeit plausible, is destined to remain such.

Chapter 3

A TRIPLE SYMBOL

The preface of this book mentions the poor attention usually paid, at least in some countries (including Italy), to the choice of a doctor's or dentist's white coat, to the extent that someone has put it on the same level as the choice of a ... shoelace.

Through an unofficial statistic, yet based on direct selling experiences, we see that a good 98% of professionals devote little or no attention to this item of clothing, usually preferring to delegate the choice to his/her staff or relativies.

Yet, among the devices that historically contributed to define the figure of the physician (stethoscope, briefcase, frontal mirror etc.), none has ever assumed such a symbolic value as the white coat, as Simona Giardina and Antonio G. Spagnolo, authors of a thorough investigation on physicians and the white coat, have highlighted. Gerhard Seeberger too has stressed this point in his presentation.

The scant attention paid to this 'insignificant' piece of clothing, however, does not mean that the role it plays in the doctor-patient relationship is disregarded. Neither, paradoxically, does the fact that some specialties (especially psychiatry, primary care medicine, pediatrics) tend to do without it mean lack of interest, as we will see shortly.

In fact, if in one of the aforesaid specialties the physician goes as far as to leave his white coat, he means to achieve a complete communication with his patient, to assure his 'compliance'. Indeed the white coat, a device judged vital for various reasons (antisepsis, tradition, obligation, habit, status symbol, external sign of knowledge and know-how) can easily be, in medical practice, an obstacle (diaphragm) to the dialogue with the patient, especially if the latter, due to his status (a minor) or condition (dementia), experiences it as such.

This detachment may lead, in many cases, to a form of anxiety, a visible reaction to the barrier, which is 'of fundamental ethical importance–scholars say–because it highlights what and how many feelings the doctor arouses in the patient with his devices.

A typical case is the so-called 'white coat hypertension' (white coat syndrome), a well-known phenomenon by virtue of which the blood pressure checkup performed by the healthcare professional in white coat causes the patient's blood pressure to increase. This, however, is avoided if the checkup is performed in a more familiar atmosphere, 'with no white sanitary uniforms around', so to speak.

A similar phenomenon is reported from veterinary medicine, where a scary-looking dog such as a mastiff, a molossus etc. begins to shake like a leaf at the sight of the white-clad veterinarian. 'In this case, however, it does not seem that the white coat is to blame', Milo Julini, a historian and long-time professor of veterinary medicine, observes, but rather a generic canine idiosyncrasy for 'all' uniforms. And also, he emphasizes, the fact that animals, perceptive as they are, better understand the attitude of those who wear the white coat. White coat hypertension, anyhow, is just one of the various sentiments underlying the doctor-patient encounter, which is historically the equivalent of what happened in the early 1800s with the introduction of the stethoscope by René Théophile Laënnec.

The device, say Spagnolo and Giardina, was initially accepted as a foreign body in the examinations of the time, which consisted in auscultation of the chest performed by placing an ear to the latter.

The estrangement between doctor and patient was not only on a physical, but also on an anthropological level (from the patient to the disease). This concept, difficult to accept at the time, is completely taken for granted today with technologized medicine, practiced remotely (telemedicine). Aside from the introspective observations illustrated by the psychologist, if we want to configure the role and therefore the values and meanings that the white coat historically assumes in the doctor-patient relationship, we come to identify, in addition to the diaphragmatic effect between doctor and patient, two further characteristics, easily perceptible to the eyes of even a distracted observer: the white coat as a status symbol and unofficial sign of knowledge and know-how.

Before examining the first characteristic, we cannot fail to note, for a sort of analogical curiosity, that the 'uniforms' of other and qualified professions or roles share the characteristics of the white coat in medicine. Who can deny, for example, that even the judge's robe, the priest's cassock or the officer's uniform, despite the different specificities, have values similar to those of the white coat? Two hints will suffice to convince ourselves that this similarity is well-funded.

In confirming the common characteristics between the white coat and the judge's robe, the President of the Court of Isernia, Enzo Di Giacomo, makes an initial distinction between the civil magistrate wearing no robe in monocratic cases and the judge of the criminal trial who, by law, must instead wear the robe. 'This obligation–explains Dr. Di Giacomo–is linked to the greater emphasis that is intended to give to the administered good (life, freedom etc.), unlike the proceedings whose object at issue is a patrimonial asset.'

In respect of the judge's robe and other uniforms there exists, also in medicine, a sort of 'white coat/no white coat' phenomenon. In the administration of law, in fact, use of the robe may decrease in an attempt to mitigate the diaphragm, an intrinsic factor common to doctors and magistrates. The President cites, by way of example, the (investigating or judging) magistrate who takes off his white coat momentarily to easily gain the confidence of a minor in a custody case, or of an interdictor in an ad hoc case or even upon assessing the violence suffered by a woman.

The ultimate goal will always be the affirmation of truth, but it will be reached more easily if the robe, the symbol of an undoubtedly strong role, is set aside to mitigate the influence of the diaphragm, a barrier that can never be completely eliminated in legal administration.

Speaking of the cassock, if the 'the cowl doesn't make the monk' saying applies to the physician, it fits even better the image and role of a clergyman, from whom the above saying explicitly draws inspiration. While admitting the presence of three factors, a learned priest such as Fr. Paolo Comba, Rector of the Collegiate Church of Santa Maria della Scala (the Cathedral) in Moncalieri (Turin) affirms that if the white coat with the cross is a compulsory status symbol for a hospital chaplain (a role he played for about ten years), in actual fact it can also be absent, without this meaning that the chaplain's role and function are diminished. The same happens in medicine, where the physician is still such, although he is not wearing a white coat. To confirm this, the Rector recalls an episode he experienced at the boarding gate of an airport. Although he was not bearing any outward sign of his priesthood, he surprisingly received a request for spiritual assistance from a passenger who was also waiting. 'I wasn't even wearing a white collar,' he points out, 'an element I've worn all the time since I was a deacon as it evokes Jesus among people. Yet that man, after realizing that I was a priest, asked me to confess him.'

Chapter 4

THE WHITE COAT CEREMONY

Society needs to distinguish people from their specific role played in the world; the cassock, therefore, like the judge's robe and the doctor's white coat, are all uniforms that 'divide' in the most literal sense of the term: they draw a demarcation line 'de visu', dividing what a person was 'before' from the one he is once he has worn the uniform.

According to the costume scholar, 'along with other details such as tabs, hats, feathers, buttons, coats of arms, colors etc., they identify various forms of authority dividing up tasks within the role. Being indicators of social meaning, they specify 'who, how and where.' The moment they are worn, the role changes as it happened with the medieval knight's armor as well as with the colours and glitters of the bullfighter uniform.

Focusing on 'white coats', as physicians are defined par excellence in journalistic language (and not only), the important meanings this polyvalent garment can assume, in this era and in the medical field, could be emblematically grasped from the so-called 'white coat ceremony', widely described by various authors thanks also to its rapid spread.

Initiated by pediatric neurologist Arnold P. Gold and his wife Sandra O. Gold, it was first held on August 20, 1993 at the Columbia University

College of Physicians & Surgeons and was repeated the following year at the Medical School of New Jersey.

A modern initiation rite, the 'Ceremony', and it is defined, has spread not only in almost all US medical faculties, but also in other parts of the world (including several European countries) as a significant moment of passage from preclinical to clinical studies.

With that celebration, future physicians are about to cross a sort of ideal bridge, as reflected in the welcome message of Nancy Angoff, dean of the Yale School of Medicine, to young people: until the first half of the bridge, young people are believed to be on the same side as their patients.

Once you've reached the halfway point, the professor admonishes, 'the language you had in common with them will gradually be replaced by the medicine language, and the sick's personal history by medical history.' Once you have reached the other end of the bridge, 'you'll be part of the medical culture,' she stresses, recommending that during the training course they should not abandon that empathy which had driven them to study medicine.

Leaving aside the various meanings that can be attributed to the event and the objections it raises (one for all, the Hippocratic oath taken 'before' and not at the end of the studies, ed.), that ceremony, on a closer inspection, can also be considered the early official acknowledgement of the white coat as the physician's main role (status symbol).

Obviously, what is meant here is not just physical dressing. Regardless of the preventive oath and other objections, 'Gold's intention–it is stressed–was to have future doctors become aware of the importance of their role at the beginning of their journey' and invite them to put on the 'virtual' white coat, the one referring to the inner dimension of each one; a white coat 'imbued with truth and reassuring words, pain-relieving gestures, awareness of one's own limits and ability to listen to the sick.'

The status symbol does not concern only the external 'façade' of the medical profession. As early as during the White Coat Ceremony, the white coat that the personalities present placed on students' shoulders to emphasise confidence in their human and professional qualities appears shorter than that of the already graduated physicians, the authors note. It is therefore a status symbol within the other.

A custom scholar remarks that in other times and circumstances, the length of this garment represented another 'role symbol'. Not many decades have passed since the length of the white coat, in hospitals and in the Faculty of Medicine, highlighted the dignity of the head physician, university lecturer or head of department.

In his 'Four in Medicine', published in the 1960s, English writer Richard Gordon describes Dr. Crate, second assistant to the all-powerful head physician Sir Lancelot (so famous he went to the hospital on a Rolls Royce driven by a chauffeur, ed.) as shining with 'very reflected light', enlivened, however, by a great privilege: he was the only one allowed to wear a white coat as long as that of the 'boss'.

At the Molinette Hospital in Turin, the largest in the region and a center of medical excellence (it would be enough to mention a few illustrious names to qualify it), the long white coat 'was a rank indicator', at least in the 70s, when Dogliotti, Biancalana, Roccia, clinicians already known for their great knowledge, became even more famous because of that 'Trial of the barons', which filled the pages of newspapers for a long time. According to the testimonies of former students, some of them, now established professionals, used to wear a longer white coat than the ordinary one.

Coming back to the significance of the Ceremony, 'as a matter of fact, the first few times one puts on the white gown, at the beginning of the profession or even as an attending student, one feels encouraged and important. Every medical student remembers that with great satisfaction.' This is what Lodovico Benso, former Full Professor of Auxology at the Faculty of Medicine, rarely white-clad like many of his pediatrician colleagues, affirms with full knowledge of the facts.

Regarding the value of the shirt/status, Benso states, with a touch of irony, that he considers it to be like a... desk. 'A place that if you are not worth it–he observes–you are not, even if you are sitting behind it. But luckily–he adds–the same statement also works the other way around'.

For Benso, the white coat status symbol seems to imply 'a hierarchy with a function in healing, which more often than not, especially in the surgical field, becomes the component of a selfish armor.' Hence his preference for the term 'role symbol.'

Depending on who wears it and how it is worn, the type of patient and the relationship established with the doctor, he admits that it can certainly be a separating factor (diaphragm) 'but not necessarily a negative one,' he stresses: a 'role touch' can also emphasize the patient's compliance.

There is a white coat for each health profession. Even at the Faculty of Veterinary Medicine there is talk of status symbols and, as at the Faculty of Medicine, wearing the white coat represented a dream and a coveted goal for students. Milo Julini, a professor of the aforesaid Faculty and now an established writer, still remembers the emotion he felt when he put it on for the first time.

However, the pet owner esteems the professional (especially when it comes to pets such as cats, dogs, hamsters etc.) not so much because the latter wears the white coat, as Carlo Girardi, former Dean of the Faculty, points out, 'but only if he demonstrates that he knows how to take care of them and how to visit them, putting them at ease without resorting to coercive maneuvers.'

'Our university masters always wore their white coats down to their knees', Ivo Zoccarato, Professor of Zooculture and member of the Italian Association for the History of Veterinary Medicine recalls. 'They inspired awe, if ever there was a need, allowing us students to recognize them immediately.'

There is another significant health analogy. Piero Maria Calcatelli, President of the Order of Pharmacists of Ancona, reminds members that the Code of Professional Conduct is not a simple statement of intent, but a set of moral and behavioral rules that professionals have freely established for themselves. In a statement dated September 2018, he emphasises that every member shall read and comply with it, and he invites members to pay attention to Article 7 on 'the professional badge and the white coat', 'although all articles have equal dignity.'

As the President explains, the article is about how a pharmacist should present himself to others and in respect of his profession. 'The white coat with the professional tag clearly visible–he observes–is the uniform that characterises him and allows whoever entering the pharmacy to identify him immediately. In fact, the patient has the right to be listened to and advised by a healthcare professional, and the pharmacy institution is chosen precisely for this reason.'

'Wearing this uniform,' he continues, 'is a guarantee for whoever steps in. What matters is not the place, but those who work there must be easily identifiable. Imagine entering a hospital and finding all the people there dressed in all sorts of ways: who would you turn to? What guarantee would you have that any person is really a healthcare provider?'

'The pharmacy being a place of health, whoever works in it must be immediately identified: we must offer a clear image–he stresses–and it is not tolerable that pharmacists present themselves to their patients in an inappropriate manner.'

Attire alone, however, is not sufficient, 'it doesn't make the monk', so to speak. A real professional must be prepared and keep up to date; that is why Article 11 refers to mandatory ongoing education. 'It is a need for any good professional, a form of respect towards others, but above all towards oneself.' 'By complying with the code and wearing the appropriate outfit, we will manage to keep the profession alive and get everyone to respect it', the President concludes.

Chapter 5

WITH OR WITHOUT A WHITE COAT?

Despite its three distinguishing factors, the white coat tends to disappear in the practice of some medical specialties, without the effective function and role of the physician being affected. The partial or total abolition of the white coat is usually justified with the specific purpose of making the therapeutic action more effective.

Francesco Colosimo, an esteemed family doctor in Rome, affirms: 'Many years ago, a young medical student was in a health clinic and had to choose a white coat to wear for his practice in the various departments. But although there were many models to choose from, he couldn't find any which fit him, none he could feel as his and could reflect what he felt he was. He thought about it and then realized that he couldn't find the white coat... because he always had it on; ever since he was a child and said that he wanted to be a doctor when he grew up, to make injections in young women's 'buttocks'. 'It's certainly not a white coat that makes a physician', adds Dr. Colosimo today. 'You, in fact, are a physician in the way you practice your profession, which I would consider a 'mission', although this term has lost its original meaning and has even become obsolete.'

'If you carry out your mission to serve the community–he adds–with that strength that you feel inside and that never makes you feel tired, if you do it with humanity, a magic word forgotten in everyday life, giving a smile and/or a caress to people who suffer, then the white coat, even if it were transparent, is there and you can see it very well.'

This does not mean to put anyone who wears it in a negative light, the doctor points out. In a hospital, for example, the white coat is indispensable; but the profession of family doctor (he stresses this term ed.), counsellor, confessor, in short, a reference point of a family, requires no rank (namely, no white coat), and the 'mission' can be carried out without a traditional garment which, in his opinion, ends up creating barriers without qualifying you.

'You are for what you do and how you do it–Dr. Colosimo emphasises–and your authority comes from this, certainly not from the white coat. Ultimately–he concludes–I still wear the white coat today, day and night. Because I am a physician and not someone who acts as a physician.' Conversely, Giovanni Vanni, a dentist in Catania, a specialist in orthodontics (or better, as he says, in dentofacial orthopedics) and author of *Doctors in the second line*, says that his relationship with the white coat has always been close and inseparable: 'Let's just say it's been my shadow', although it wasn't quite like that at first. Unaccustomed to that uniform, he sometimes forgot to wear it, until one day, at the postgraduate school, the director reproved him good-naturedly, saying that 'a doctor without a white coat is like a driver without a license.'

'Since then', he continues, 'the white coat and I have become one.' When he happens to find himself sharing a clinical opinion with a colleague, 'I feel I'm missing something essential without my shadow', he says. For him, a white coat is not only a symbol, but, like his father–also a doctor–he deems it a necessary device for his work. He wears a freshly laundered one every day 'for my dignity', he points out, but above all out of respect for the patient as well as for hygienic purposes. And for fear of finding himself without a washed and ironed white coat, he has a huge number of summer and winter garments on hand.

He gets angry and can hardly control himself when he sees some colleagues walking to the bar wearing a white coat. He also gets very annoyed and ashamed when he sees someone else wearing a dirty white coat. At the postgraduate school, when he noticed that someone in his absence had taken possession of his white coat and hung it up stained in the locker, he preferred to skip class rather than wear it.

Speaking of white coats, he recalls an episode in a dental clinic caused by a distraction he defines 'proverbial' and still makes him smile. Having failed to notice that he was wearing his colleague Mirella's white coat instead of his own, he came across numerous smiles for which he couldn't find a reason. Only when a colleague greeted him, in a falsetto voice, 'good morning, doctor' did he understand what he had done.

Also uncertain on whether a doctor should wear a white coat is psychogeriatrician Luigi Pernigotti: 'The smart patient appreciates use of the white coat. So when the visit involves touching a patient, the latter appreciates that the doctor uses a hygienic device.' He admits, however, that the smart patient also appreciates that the doctor takes it off when the visit only requires to be close to the patient without touching him.

If, on the one hand, diaphragm implies a role of authoritative counselor, on the other hand the white coat serves to identify the person in uniform who has the social task of making you feel good, he comments. At that moment, one moves from the diaphragm to a device of social proximity. The bottom line is that if there are different ways to wear the white coat, the physician should know how to adopt them depending on the patient's need. Psychiatry is also one of the specialties that often does without a white coat, authoritative Pier Maria Furlan, former Professor of Psychiatry, Dean of Faculty and Vice-Chancellor at the University of Turin, confirms. In explaining the reasons, he dwells on some historical data: 'Only after the mid-1900s in Italy–he says–did we get to the point of considering hospital and asylum doctors on the same level. Only then was the white coat considered a category identification item.'

Although the white coat remains mandatory for the existence of psychiatric wards in hospitals (following the anti-asylum movements, the greater importance given to social and therapeutic displacement from asylums), it nevertheless appears anachronistic to many, who regard it even a symbol of biological oppression in antithesis to social recovery.

'In the healthcare field, the white coat, and attire itself, are a message not only for patients, but also for relatives, the public and healthcare personnel'–he says. 'And given the variety of situations, it is mainly up to the psychiatrist to develop a message tailored for the patient's conditions.' Today more than ever, and despite unity of vision declarations, various conceptions of pathology and treatment dominate in psychiatry. For the biologic-somatic view, characterised by pharmacological interventions, the white coat is a privileged distinguishing instrument.

According to the rehabilitative-social view, it is a contradiction in terms (oxymoron), while for the psychotherapeutic view, it should be treated as a cause-effect of what the patient feels. In psychiatry, however, the white coat is not always an element of reassurance nor a guarantee toward the patient and his needs, as is the case in other healthcare disciplines. 'Whether you like it or not (like Furlan, ed.), medical practice contains a custodial social mandate.' Therefore, he would add a fourth distinguishing factor to the other three (diaphragm, status symbol, index of knowledge and know-how): the sign of the social control mandate inherent in psychiatry itself. The effect on the patient should be part of the elaboration of the relationship, 'because wearing the white coat or not'–he says–'is always a sort of statement of intent.'

Chapter 6

FROM STARS ...

After seeing the two opposite 'dressing situations'–wearing or not wearing a white coat–we cannot but focus on a third one, which we will call the 'near-white coat'. Before, however, we need to briefly mention a medical therapy called 'clown therapy', which is officially based on smiling. The patient smiles; so do those who see such therapy being practiced and sometimes the therapist himself, though in a different way.

Clown therapy became greatly popular all over the world mainly thanks to a tragicomic movie of 1998, 'Patch Adams', based on the life of the therapy's founder, Hunter Doherty 'Patch' Adams, whose role was performed by Robin Williams, an eclectic, brilliant actor. However, the clown therapy he had brilliantly illustrated in the movie was not enough to keep him from taking his life when he learnt that dementia was hanging over him.

Opposed from the outset by the academic medical establishment, this therapy was initially labelled as an at least 'peculiar' technique, a rather euphemistic, infinitely finer term if compared to 'waiting room clown', a nickname given to Patch Adams and his followers which later turned into a non-denigrating one. Evidence of that are the countless awards conferred on its founder (among which an honorary degree in Pedagogy, conferred on him in 2007 by the University of Bologna ed.).

The 'Adams' recipe' to treat the body and mind includes entertainment and smiling. This is nothing new, because since the dawn of medicine, both have always been regarded a healthy coefficient. Dr. Hunter 'Patch' Adams puts them on the same level as love, believing that humor is an actual antidote for all ills. 'At the end of the day, when people are asked what they like of life–he says–what matters is the fun they get out of it'.

Chemistry supports these affirmations: for, as general research highlights, smiling favors the secretion of natural chemical substances capable of generating sensations of brightness and well-being.

This is obviously not the right occasion and place to delve into the chemical and psychological mechanisms which are believed to make that practice efficient. What is of interest here is the role played by the white coat in the physician/clown relationship with its 'clown therapy patient'– let us call him this way, if anything, to distinguish him from others.

Getting back to the examination of the white coat's three main psychosociological factors identified earlier (diaphragm, status symbol, sign of knowledge and know-how), we cannot fail to observe that out of the three factors, only two co-exist in the light of clown therapy.

The first factor, that is, the barrier between physician and patient, is deliberately cancelled by the 'clown doctor' to break down any communication obstacle with a patient that in most cases is a child (but the same is true for other sick patients) who is often intimidated by such barrier. Otherwise, there is no compliance at all.

If the clown doctor's white coat tears down the barrier of distrust and fear the child generally feels towards the physician (in this case there's no diaphragm anymore), 'there remains the fact that for all adults and children, that physician is not a clown, but a physician dressed as clown', Franco Prono, professor of Italian film making at Turin-based DAMS, affirms.

However, it is also true that the image of the white coat as a status symbol contrasting with the clown image tends to get blurred. But that would be just an impression fostered by the noble, therapeutic goal which drove the physician to 'dress up' in that way. His choice, in fact, strengthens rather than opposes the idea of the white coat being a status symbol, since paradoxically it also reinforces the external meaning of knowledge and know-how.

After all, he is a medical researcher trying other paths (and kinds of attire) to achieve his therapeutic targets more easily. The clown therapist of Patch Adams, therefore, does not cease to wear his white coat; he just transforms it to reduce its 'diaphragmatic charge' and make his 'therapy' more efficient.

A question arises from the reference to Patch Adams: what kind of impact has the white coat itself and its contents (especially its role in the doctor-patient relationship) had on the film world?

Beginning with the successful film directed by Tom Shadyac (1998), probably even the least careful cinephile has not missed the final scene. It's the scene in which young Hunter Adams, after overcoming various banishments and the establishment's die-hard distrust toward his smiling therapy, leaves the stage where he has just been solemnly declared doctor and deliberately shows his... buttock to the audience. What ensues is an immediate closeup of the faces of a bewildered public, utterly upset by that 'unacademic' image.

In fact, at that moment Adams is not wearing the white coat reserved to the new doctor he has just been declared, but the black robe of the graduate-to-be, as is customary in the US. But even if he were already white-clad as his senior colleagues, he wouldn't probably give up staging the same performance, his nonconformist nature being such as to drive him to turn into a clown for the love of the patient.

Patch Adams will not get as far as to peel off his gown (not his robe) to uncover his butt, but he will not hesitate to dye his face or wear a fake red nose to carry out his 'therapeutic revolution'.

Therefore, beginning with the doctor as a frequent (co)-protagonist of film history, we have attempted to trace, with the help of a few scholars, the ways in which the doctor expresses himself, directly or indirectly, through his white coat and its inherent contents.

Let us take for example the well-known *NHS doctor* by Luigi Zampa (1968), which paved the way, the following year, for the equally successful *Prof. Dr. Guido Tersilli, head physician of Villa Celeste, a clinic affiliated with the NHS*, a movie directed by Luciano Salce and featuring a character impeccably performed by Alberto Sordi.

In the film, Dr. Tersili, like a general before his white-clad troops, shows off an immaculate, fluttering white coat on the notes of Piero Piccioni's *Aesculapius March*. How can one fail to see, in that musical piece, which could be defined a 'triumphal white-clad walk', a praise of the status symbol (more than the know-how and the diaphragm, also present in the background), that is, an overt display of professional medical pride?

Nothing more different from the pompous image of Dr. Terzilli can be found in another famous series, *ER Doctors on the front line*, where the white coat worn in an emergency room is visibly stressed, wrinkled, worn out by extreme use. It is like the image of a faded pride we find in a 2001 series that proved to be a milestone; it even changed its name commonly used, from hospital uniform to 'scrub' (relating to the scrubbing of hands and forearms before a surgery).

This series shows physicians wearing short-sleeved uniforms under a long-sleeved T-shirt, also on the home-work route. Finally, when it comes to our days, in *Dr. House*, a latest series focused on medical research, the main character does not use the white coat, which is, on the contrary, worn impeccably by his staff.

If you look at it through its usual garment, the image of the doctor in cinematography, from the 80s onwards, appears changed. From the famous fiction *Scrubs*, where the shirt practically disappears replaced by a short-sleeved jacket on a T-shirt with long sleeves, to the equally famous series of *Dr. House*. The dark Hugh Laurie, doctor not empathetic, but brilliant, always and strictly in civilian clothes, contrasts with the image of his staff, all impeccable in their fresh shirts ironing. Whether worn or not, paradoxically the message that reaches the patient does not change: you shouldn't judge a book by its cover

Chapter 7

...TO STARLETS

'How do people usually address you? By your rank or by your title of doctor? What do you prefer?' A medical officer is often asked such questions, at least according to what the interested parties say.

Luigi De Meo, a (retired) army colonel of the 'Taurinense' Alpine Brigade and a urology specialist with missions in Iraq (Kurdistan), Albania, Mozambique, Bosnia-Herzegovina, Kosovo and Afghanistan behind him, explains: 'Normally, military staff and, unexpectedly, ordinary citizens too address me by my rank rather than by my title of doctor. I personally prefer and am proud of that: I deem the fact that civilians call me by my rank a sign of respect towards institutions.'

Less frequent, albeit similarly inspired, is the question of 'white coat wearability'. In down-to-earth, though clearly metaphorical terms: how does a military doctor wear the white coat? Over or under the uniform? To put it simply: does the uniform or the white coat come first?

De Meo has no doubt: 'Unfortunately, almost all military doctors wear it 'over' the uniform, since 'official physicians' are the majority, while 'medical officers' who wear it under the uniform are really numbered. De Meo is proud to be part of it because, as he says: 'I also tried to honor my oath putting unreserved respect for duty before self-interest.'

On the prevalence of one over the other, De Meo reiterates: 'In my humble opinion, the white coat should never prevail over the uniform. Being a medical officer is a free life choice which involves being faithful to the oath of practicing medicine 'to the best of one's knowledge and belief', always bearing in mind one's own duties, fundamental values and respect of constitutional principles.'

Federico Lunardi, a colonel and urgency medicine specialist, with service experience in Bosnia, Afghanistan, Somalia and Antarctica, as well as an esteemed author of several publications, has a more nuanced view: 'Uniform and white coat blend together', he says. 'The sick soldier, like the civilian we give assistance to, is not interested in the external content, but in listening and how we take care of him. Besides, if the white coat reveals 'cleanliness', the military uniform indicates values and ideals.'

As for the possible prevalence of one over the other, 'I had to face borderline situations–he recalls–when, after being involved into fire actions by hostile people, I needed to think more of my military training than my health profession. After all, even the firefighter, before entering a burning house, wonders if collapse is imminent or if he has the time and way to save human lives.'

In your experience, have there been any uncertain circumstances as to which one should prevail–the white coat or uniform?–'I'd answer there haven't', he says. 'The institution asks us to take care of the military men entrusted to us, not only by healing them if they are sick, but also contributing to the maintenance of their health with all possible hygienic indications. Historically, hygiene has its roots on the battlefield, where it is necessary to preserve the combatant's health.'

Leaving aside for a moment the question of whether the white coat is worn over or under the uniform, how does the 'civilian' patient see the military doctor? And does the uniformed patient also see the civilian doctor differently? The impression is that the civilian patient certainly sees the uniformed doctor with different eyes and, to some extent, with admiration and respect as well. Others look at the doctor with complancency, underestimating his preparation and professional competence.

However, the same could be said for the military patient who, considering the doctor in uniform a less capable professional insofar as he does not meet his requirements and/or expectations, mistakenly perceives a greater preparation and professionalism in the civilian doctor.

'However, this is a challenging answer, especially in the image society we live in', Lunardi points out. 'Sometimes there are short-sighted or distorted views due to preconceptions or rigid mental schemes. They usually last until you find yourself working together (alongside colleagues) or in the "dual" doctor-patient relationship (if you are with the sick person).'

Many soldiers,' Lunardi admits, 'have the prejudice that the hospitalist is always better prepared than the military doctor. But after sharing the weight of the backpack (just to quote Bedeschi's words), the military doctor sometimes ends up being idealised by his own soldiers.'

To clarify the figure of and the consideration about the two professionals, it is worth reflecting on which of the three dominant characteristics of the white coat is judged prevalent. De Meo says: 'Certainly (I hope so), the external sign of knowledge and know-how.'

In more practical terms, this involves demonstrating, with one's professionalism, skills and behavior, that one is worthy of the uniform, rank and role and of the importance of the medical officer's figure, also in civil society.

Lunardi agrees but fears the inevitable fall into the category of the 'Master of those who know'. 'All of us reveal and demonstrate our human and professional depth when we find ourselves acting in the most remote places', he observes. 'Two stitches applied while kneeling, with a headlight illuminating the unfortunate person in the middle of the woods, does not increase the status symbol, creates unity and, above all, leaves a sense of gratitude in the rescued soldier no medal can ever be comparable to.'

Chapter 8

YOU CANNOT JUDGE A BOOK BY ITS COVER

'They're beautiful jackets, of unsurpassable quality, perfectly wearable, looking stylish and professional, made of a soft and long-lasting material.' These are the enthusiastic words with which Dr. Nick Karney, an endodontist in Philadelphia (USA), wrote to the company that makes his professional jackets and gowns, congratulating them for 'decisively' putting him in a new, more pleasant light in the eyes of his patients. We quote the most significant parts of his letter which appear to be in contrast with the highly provocative title of this chapter, as if to explode the truth of a proverb common to several languages. This is followed by an equally enthusiastic email of an English woman doctor from Wigan, a town halfway between Liverpool and Manchester. She is aware of being considered–and seeing herself–more attractive professionally when wearing a certain white coat model.

'Before practicing in a rather wealthy area of Philadelphia, where patients treated me with that deference and respect that are usually owed to a dental specialist, I had practiced medicine in a little town north of the State of New York, where patients were of a completely different kind.

Besides being patients, they were friends of the GP they had probably seen for a long time: in fact, they openly showed their perplexity before any other dental specialist taking care of their mouth.

Seeing how they watched me approach the dentist chair to perform a root canal, I immediately realised they didn't trust me, a young endodontics specialist. Maybe because I was young, or they didn't know me so they were fearful, and it wasn't that general fear that assails every patient before the drill.

To be honest, before I put on one of your jackets, they didn't trust me, also because of my white coat, which looked definitely horrible, and my general look, which wasn't at all professional.

I can't say how many times a patient asked me if I had ever performed the surgery I was about to carry out; or whether he was the first to undergo it, or even whether I knew what I was doing. Not to mention the many anxious phone calls I received from suffering patients during and owing to the post-surgery period.

Now, instead, some months after I started wearing your white coat, it is incredible to see the different way patients watch me moving about in the operating room, aware of the (also financial) value of what I am doing.

Very few patients ask me how old I am and, above all, whether I have any experience with that surgery. Meanwhile the anxious phone calls I used to receive after the operation have gradually decreased.

Hence my profound conviction that the intense post-surgical pain is not so much due to the patient's real suffering as to the idea he's got of his surgeon's experience or to his fear of him. Yet I can assure you that my approach to the patient has not changed at all. It's just that we live in a society which is ready to judge and is prone to finding something to criticise about. Conversely, the professional look suggested by the model I'm wearing gratifies the physician wearing it with an immediate wink and smug appreciation.'

Contrary to the popular saying 'You cannot judge a book by its cover' Nina Bal Gourgey, an odontologist in Wigam (GB), says that the white coat is of great importance. 'For it is after all the first impression patients receive when they meet me. It is as if I handed them a "living" business card.'

But there is more to it. 'Dressing "properly"–adds Dr. Gourgey–has also an incredible impact on how I feel: professional, attractive, female. I feel that I'm conveying the image of a trustworthy professional without having to give up my femininity.'

Thanks to this first immediate perception and the role the white coat plays in nonverbal communication, Dr. Gourgey concludes by saying that a 'right' white coat surely plays an important role in the interpersonal relationship with the patient. It is the same conclusion other qualified studies and testimonies come to, by virtue of which if the white coat doesn't make the doctor, it would anyhow make the physician, albeit partially; even in intensive care units. Let us examine some of such studies in chronological order.

A study published in 2013, carried out by the University of Calgary (Canada) on 337 family members visiting a relative of theirs in an intensive care unit showed that most of them tended to rely more on properly dressed doctors, wearing white coats or hospital uniforms. And what is more (a very important detail!), the tag on the chest, with easy-to-read name and title.

It also turned out that the physician, whether in a blue or grey suit and tie, or in a casual suit, doesn't give a good impression, as it seems more difficult to hypothesise in him reassuring virtues like competence, honesty, commitment, and up-to-date professional preparation.

The research confirmed, even in more critical units like First Aid, greater reliability resulting from physicians' traditional attire.

Hence the conclusion drawn by the Canadian researchers: like the emotional importance of placebo in drug trials, physicians, especially in emergency and intensive care units, should also be able to inspire esteem from the start. For it is right here, where relatives of endangered patients and physicians meet for the first time, that an atmosphere of immediate trust should be established.

The article on the Calgary investigation, written by Serena Zoli, a former journalist of Corriere della Sera, and referred to in July 2018 in the *Magazine* journal of Fondazione Umberto Veronesi, examines another study made public by the University of Michigan, which will widely be described in the following chapter.

Chapter 9

DOES THE WHITE COAT DEFINE A DOCTOR?

An investigation on 4,000 patients, carried out in Michigan and published by *BMJ Open*, was intended to verify the impact of physician attire on trust and treatment. Patients were asked to view 14 pictures of men and women wearing different types of physician attire, from casual to very formal clothes.

Asked directly on how physicians should dress, 44% of the interviewees opted for formal attire plus the white coat, and 26% for the hospital device plus the white coat. As for first aid surgeons and physicians, the uniform alone got 34% of votes followed by the uniform-attire combination (23%). On such occasion, half of the interviewees highlighted the importance of attire, while a third even stated that patients' satisfaction with treatment would be influenced by it.

Commenting on the investigation, the curator, Professor Christopher Petrilli, of the School of Medicine of the University, stated that while the importance of professional attire at Wall Street, in Courts, or in any other field of activity is quite clear and indicative, the dress code in medicine is varied: 'We physicians should pay attention to the level of professionalism reflected on our attire and take into account the patient's wishes'.

The investigation found that every patient, consciously or unconsciously, would like to tell his own doctor 'I evaluate from your way of style if I can trust you or not.' As underlined by journalist Serena Zoli (see previous chapter), who published this investigation in Italy for the Umberto Veronesi Foundation, this is especially true at the first meeting, when we don't yet have a clear understanding of the credentials of the doctor who has our health in his hands.

A similar investigation was conducted by the department of epidemiology of Universitaet Spital Zuerich (USZ), the university hospital of Zurich: it involved 834 patients, who answered a questionnaire after viewing the pictures of a physician in various clothing combinations.

The investigation revealed that physicians should wear a white coat instead of coloured dresses; this is not just for a question of taste, but for the impact on the success of treatments: 'Patients, in fact, do not open themselves up to a physician who's not very formally dressed, while they tend to follow less strictly instructions and guidelines provided by physicians in casual attire.'

The declared objective of the investigation was not to reveal what appears pleasant in patients' eyes, but rather to ascertain their (mostly unconscious) reaction to the physician's appearance. A third of the interviewees deem the physician's look very important, while about 25% think that attire also influences the opinion on treatment (the same result obtained by the Michigan investigation).

The outfit most trusted by patients always includes the white coat, preferably accompanied by clothes of this colour. As Hugo Sax, Head of Department at the Zurich Hospital, explains, the research indicates 'which attire inspires trust, in which outfit physicians appear more accessible and helpful; and, above all, if patients attribute professional skills to a certain type of attire.'

The role played by the white coat appears unique when a patient is frail. Since the handicapped person, who is not subject to the schemes imposed by the adult age, has a more childlike, sensitive view, the (unprecedented) study on the white coat and disability started by SIOH, the Italian Society of Odontostomatology for Handicap, is indeed significant and original.

This Society was founded in 1985 by 'enlightened dentists', as *Odontoiatria33* defined them in a 2016 article. They had the professional and human intuition to understand before others the importance of organising for the disabled a scientific society of 'special scrubs' for equally special patients like those with various disabilities–physical, sensory, intellectual, mental, medical, emotional, and/or social.

This is not an 'oceanic investigation' since it was carried out in the restricted area of slightly less than 300 disabled people and their caregivers; however, it is an enlightening contribution to learn how both the disabled and the caregivers experience the relationship with the coat worn by the dentists treating them.

Before delving into the details of the study, let us hear how the healers live their relationship with the white coat. Dr. Fausto Assandri, visiting professor at the State University of Milan as well as medical director of the Complex Unity of Maxillofacial Surgery–Odontology of the Polyclinic and SIOH president, says: 'We, as a "special dentists", when we get to the clinic, we put on a white coat first thing in the morning. If patients see us simple and plain-clothes, they sometimes do not even recognise us and consequently do not greet us. Because without the white coat... they simply cannot see us.'

Aside from patients' reaction, putting on a white coat as first act of the day 'is a form of respect for ourselves and others, of awareness of our role and duties', Assandri points out. But it is also an honor, an act of great symbolic value: 'I strip myself of what I was before and now I'm totally devoted to others... to my "neighbour"', he says.

If medicine is a 'non-exact' science, it is precisely because it is (or should be) imbued with the value of solidarity, having only two true goals: to relieve pain and save other people's lives. Wearing a white coat, therefore, 'means having the knowledge and know-how in respect of science and conscience. But if the doctor is unable to love "his neighbour", he will never be a good physician nor an odontologist.'

These expressions give rise to the immediate, persuasive conviction that dentistry for the disabled, 'special' as it is, is not a job for everyone. This is indirectly confirmed by the code of ethics stating that 'in the reciprocal doctor-patient alliance... the caring relationship is fundamental.'

As Elena Pozzani, specialist in orthognathodontics, visiting professor at the University of Padua and a dynamic National Secretary of SIOH, remarks, the recent Covid-19 pandemic has disrupted the pathways of prevention and dental care for the disabled, but even worst, for the 'special dentists', who perhaps have been committed for years to turn an uncooperative patient into an ideal one. Seeing him dressed like the staff dealing with nasopharyngeal swabs, many of those patients have been hit again by anxiety of the dentist's chair.

Chapter 10

YOU CAN TELL A COUNTRY BY ITS MEDICAL UNIFORM

To understand, therefore, the impact of the 'white coat look of special dentists', a short questionnaire was administered to 136 disabled people (aged between 6 and 25), who were basically asked what their favorite colour was; but above all, if they were afraid of the dentist.

As many caregivers (aged between 22 and 36) were asked which feeling (confidence or anxiety) was caused by the white colour, if they considered white the 'ideal' colour or at least the 'most professional' one among others. The odd result, Pozzani comments, is that 30% of patients prefer the yellow colour, 52% even the dentist dressed in blue, while 88% (incredible!) are not at all afraid of the dentist.

Predictably, the reactions of caregivers are different: 80% of them say the white coat inspires confidence, while 38% consider it the ideal colour, as opposed to 23%, who consider blue ideal. White is deemed more professional by 62%, as opposed to 12% who attribute such quality to green and a minimal 2% who opt for blue. A solid 24%, however, believe (perhaps more justifiably, ed.) that the colour of the scrubs has nothing to do with the physician's professionalism.

At that moment, in order to focus on a few points, we asked a few questions to both organizers of this short, unprecedented investigation, which will be followed by a more extensive one shortly. In any case, this original investigation among individuals with such different disabilities does not obscure the question as to why it was conducted in parallel among their caregivers as well. Are they the first interpreters of their patients' feelings and moods?

'Dealing mainly with patients in developmental age–says Assandri–I found essential to involve their parents in the questionnaire, because a child goes by instinct in choosing people, places and situations, while it is the parent who rationalises and makes choices for his children.'

The same is true for an adult with a deficit: 'The guardian/administrator chooses the treatment paths and expresses the necessary consents to activate the therapeutic paths', Pozzani adds.

This is not all. If the variety of colours indicated by the disabled is amazing, what is also surprising is that there is no reference to the white colour, which is widely known to be the most common one throughout the world. Yellow is mentioned, blue is indicated, but no hint is given of white. If most of the patients preferred coloured scrubs, why this unexpected predilection for yellow?

'Because it is the color of sunshine, light and positivity. This could suggest that they are "happy" in life, but also in the dental clinic, where the questions were asked.' A vibrant colour, the two experts add, can activate positive stimuli in such patients because their cognitive pathways are instinctive, not blocked by mental preconceptions of an educational and ethical nature.

Anyhow, 52% of the disabled indicate blue as their favorite colour. The reason for 'this' choice could be that most of the overcoats used over the last two years are blue/light blue. Regardless of the colour preferences that emerged from the mini survey, it seems clear to both researchers that the value of the white coat in healthcare remains 'universal' because of the message of hygiene, purity, and disinfection it conveys.

Another doubt: if the 'special' dentist didn't wear any scrubs, how could the disabled person react? 'Actually, in the pre-Covid era, I sometimes chose to wear plain clothes when I had to visit an uncooperative child for the first time, just to remove an obstacle to the caring relationship–Assandri recalls–then Covid came along and changed everything.' 'Wearing scrubs, even double scrubs–Pozzani confirms–has become imperative to protect us professionals, but also our patients, from cross-infections. In this respect, I dare say that every cloud has a silver lining!'

Finally (and surprisingly), the investigation highlighted that 88% are not afraid of the dentist, while non-disabled people (caregivers and others) are. Doesn't that sound a bit strange? 'Treating disabled, often uncooperative patients implies, mainly on an outpatient level, an often long "desensitisation" process. The greatest satisfaction of our work lies not so much in dental care as in making a patient cooperative and overcome dental phobia.'

The enthusiastic letters of the previous chapter, but also the result of the three investigations, provide the inspiration to mention the role played by the white coat in the look of professionals from various countries. In other words: if medicine is one but there are various ways to practice it, is the same true for the attire the physician must (or can) wear at various latitudes?

An investigation on the shapes and colours, but above all the 'way' the doctor lives his white coat has yielded surprising results. It is true that there is a different doctor uniform in every nation since habits and styles change significantly from country to country.

As a matter of fact, four big types of attire can be identified around the world: the 'basic attire', widespread in central Europe, the United

States and Oceania, where a simple, economical suit or simply a white coat is used; the 'comfortable attire' of Northern Europe and Italy which involve tunic and trousers, as comfort is considered essential.

In France, Spain, Portugal, Russia, the former republics of the USSR and in all the Middle East, physicians and dentists are considered 'elegant': in such countries, in fact, uniqueness and the search for elegance come first and can indifferently include a tunic/trousers suit but also a skirt or scrubs, albeit used as dress. Finally, the 'exclusive attire' used in Asian countries and South America, where every physician prefers to have a specific image, as different as possible from his colleagues.

A last note of aesthetic and social nature is dedicated to white, the most popular colour, which has become traditional since the late nineteenth century with the inclusion of scientific principles into medical practice replacing the formal black colour, largely used earlier.

If tradition sees in white the dominant colour mainly for hygienic reasons, peacefully acquired, and as a symbol of the medical profession, which colours would gradually be replacing it today, at least within some branches?

White remains by far the most popular colour, although statistics show that the area, the medical specialisation, and the type of clinic, whether private or state-run, are also very important for the prevalence of colour. In the Anglo-Saxon countries, for example, black and dark grey are mainly required, while in Eastern Europe, the Middle East and Asia, white and possibly classic, subtle colours such as light blue, light green etc. stand out. In South America, white is the prevailing colour, except in the field of aesthetic surgery.

On the other hand, Latin countries such as Italy, Spain and France are more alternative; they tend to follow the chromatic indications coming from fashion and use all the rainbow' colours.

Chapter 11

THE NOBLE VOICE OF ITALIAN DENTISTRY

According to Carlo Guastamacchia, a noble voice of Italian dentistry, the public image of whoever practices dentistry at any level is that of an individual at the top of social position and responsibility, an image that must therefore be rigorously expressed and maintained also (and especially) in respect of attire. It is a real 'uniform', as defined by the prestigious opinion leader, that identifies and represents such important role. Equally essential to him is the recommendation, mainly addressed to his younger colleagues, to never appear 'in plain clothes' to the patient.

In addition to hygiene issues, not appearing 'in uniform' is inspired by a misunderstood sense of familiarity that has nothing to do with the moment of professional practice. The worst occurs when some young colleague, out of a supposed sense of youthful nonchalance, shows up before the patient with jeans pierced at the knee, frayed or curiously multicolored. Also 'Sports' shirts too are not in line with proper, due professional presentations.

The key, he points out, is immediate professional identification, since each person working in the office must be easily recognisable by name and role. It is obviously vital that the dentist presents above all himself with his name and surname as well as a white coat which will, therefore, bear the same distinguishing elements well in view.

In some countries, it is common for a patient to be greeted by a dentist wearing a uniform with the logo or symbol of the university where he graduated well printed on it. This is an odd custom, at least for Italy. It does not seem to be common here–he observes–even though communicating where one studied and graduated should be a reason for justified pride. This is even more important these days, since a real ranking exists that places each university in positions of greater or lesser importance.

As for professional clothing–he comments–there are no specific rules to date, neither on a national nor a European level. Some recommendations only suggest the constant use of a white coat or similar items to cover the clothes that are normally used in external routes. Here are some of Guastamacchia's personal suggestions, starting from the principles inspiring this topic:

- Every collaborator must have his white coat with his name, at chest height, written clearly so that it can be read easily from a conversational distance. Next to it must also appear the title. In this regard, Guastamacchia deems magnetic adhesive tags particularly useful, as they spare the hassle of rewriting the job title each time the uniform is changed.
- It is advisable to call the hygienist by the name preceded by the title (e.g., Dr. Maria) to distinguish him/her from the dentist. The patient, in fact, needs the two professionals to be distinct and identifiable in their specific duties and responsibilities.
- Contrary to popular opinion, it is not essential that all uniforms be white. Collaborators may be free to have colors of their liking, as long as they are plain and not patterned. On the other hand,

uniforms in violent colors such as orange, deep red or yellow should be excluded being perceived as 'not very reassuring'.

- Still about white, a non-binding but indicative criterion could be to identify the different rules inside the clinic using different colors. This is not, however, a peremptory suggestion, he specifies.
- The traditional white coat can be replaced by a more comfortable uniform consisting of trousers and jacket, preferably with pockets. For female dentists, hygienists and dental assistants, trousers and jacket are always preferable to the skirt because they are never embarrassing in any posture and positioning, he stresses.
- There are special cases of dental assistants working in pedodontic practices: to gain the admiration of children, their white coats (appropriately?) show magnetically applied wings that simulate the appearance of angels or butterflies. 'These are very personal choices,' he comments, 'which are not to be considered indispensable in any practice where children are treated.'
- As for pockets, a dentist should have two of them at chest height; sleeves should be long, when they serve to mask any tattoos, which, albeit not objectionable on a personal level–he notes–cannot be considered irreproachable with regard to the image and role of the health worker. Same goes for any type of personal ornament, from bracelets to earrings, necklaces, piercings of various kinds. Footwear, however, should always consist of surgical clogs with a safety lace, preferably in the rear.

Last but not least, a further observation. Those who practice a lot of dental surgery and/or implantology are accustomed to considering non-woven fabric disposable gowns made of propylene or assimilated substances. Obviously, whether disposable or not, every gown must look absolutely clean: any speck, even the smallest, must immediately suggest washing the 'contaminated' part: in fact, the image of the surgeon or dentist appearing more appreciable by stains indicating his industriousness has definitively disappeared.

The closure of the white coat or jacket can be made with zippers or buttons, depending on personal choice. Plain clothes are not allowed– says Guastamacchia, reiterating the ban mentioned at the beginning. Even the dental technician, if admitted by the dentist in the operating room to help with prosthetic adjustments, must wear a proper 'uniform'. He must never appear in plain clothes.

Chapter 12

'UNDER THE WHITE COAT'

Stefano Almini, a dental technician in Brescia, mainly known for having been a member of the ECM National Commission for years, is a lover of dentistry and culture. A lecturer in various Italian cities, with this testimony he reveals himself to be a careful observer of the changes that have occurred in recent times in the relationship with the patient and in the dentist's professional attire.

The title of this chapter refers to a film by Carlo Vanzina, which was an epoch-making event in the '80s because it recounted the world of fashion shows, coveted by aspiring models for the spotlight and the over-the-top lifestyle.

A very 'social' movie, we would say today; but also an alienating one, the expression of a reality lacking in authentic values: beautiful women on the catwalks with unaffordable dresses, but with a problem: underneath the dress they had... nothing. It is exactly the contrary to what happens with the white coat, whatever it is or represents, Almini says.

He asks himself: since the Order a health professional belongs to is composed of two Bars (physicians and dentists), is their white coat the same or different? The two professionals share the same Order and dignity, but the roles of the doctor and the dentist are operationally different, because the white coat worn in a ward is not the same as that worn in a dental office.

In the first case it is long, with vertical buttons on the front and an open collar in jacket style, also allowing a shirt with or without a tie.

The way of working, on the other hand, has changed the dentist's white coat over time. Specialised in Odontostomatology with a medical background, the dentist of the second half of twentieth century rarely worked sitting: he stood, bent over the patient, in a position that was certainly uncomfortable, alongside a nurse who had no specific dental skills or duties. His white coat was long and buttoned, he used it also when he had to intervene as a dentist, serving as a public health physician.

The arrival of the degree in dentistry and the ergonomic applications developed over the years by incomparable Carlo Guastamacchia involved the acquisition of a new professional identity, as a pure odontologist. From that moment, a slow metamorphosis began, based on the new job positions.

In the '70s, a new element made its appearance in the practice: the dentist's chair. The dentist began to work in a seated position while the assistant, in the early days, remained standing alongside the 'doctor' who, thanks to the new wheelchair, could glide quickly from the dental unit to the mobile cabinet.

According to the European ISO 6385* rule, the white coat began to shorten from its former length: in fact, nothing could be more uncom-

* *It is the standard that establishes the basic principles of ergonomics as a guideline for the design of work systems by defining the relevant basic terms. It also describes an integrated approach to work system design in which ergonomists cooperate with other subjects involved in design and attention is paid to human, technical, and social requirements in a balanced manner throughout the process.*

fortable than sitting in a wheelchair and having to move a lever with a foot to activate the turbines. For dentists, as we know, use not only their hands but also their feet; the white coat, therefore, had to adapt to this function.

In the meantime, the patient also changed position–another epoch-making change–becoming more and more reclined on the back of the dental unit. The arrival of the dentist's chair, and of the assistant soon afterwards, was accompanied by a change in the patient's posture: less sitting and more leaning.

Since the dentist often worked four-handedly with his assistant, both sitting side by side, the dentist's uniform 'had' to include fairly comfortable trousers, not too tight so as not to hinder the movement of the foot when activating the dental unit's turbines and above all not to create any discomfort during the long hours spent in that position. And under the trousers, a mythical medical heritage, a white clog was used in various ways and shapes.

Minimalistic gowns

Let us take a closer look at that dentist's evolving white coat. In the '80s and '90s it had a pocket on the left capable of representing, albeit in a small space, a valuable content, evocative of history and mystery. The pocket of the head physician's white coat could contain pens, pencils, the pass to 'swipe' his presence, the card for the coffee machine: all objects for a forgotten semeiotics, such as the phonendoscope.

In the dental field, the upper left pocket of the doctor's white coat has undergone a metamorphosis becoming a dentist's white coat breast pocket. The '80s white coat could still proudly bear items such as the dental probe and mirror pair, strictly unbagged and unsterilised. A respectable dentist would not have been allowed to go from one dental unit to another (almost all offices had at least two) with a white coat without a pocket.

A forgotten companion of many visits to a patient totally entrusted to his dentist without the obsessions of today, the pocket is disappearing slowly and quietly, moving away from the customs of the past. The mirror and probe still exist, but they are separate, sterilised, lying in the drawer before being placed, at the right moment, on the examination kit.

The breast pocket of the past was the witness of a dentistry without too many procedures, perhaps unaware of the risks of infection, but certainly more 'livable', sheltered from the stress that characterises today's daily life. Attempts to make the white coat as cleanable and as less a receptacle as possible are making it more 'minimalist': along with the breast pocket, in fact, its 'sister pockets', inevitably considered potential receptacles for bacteria, are disappearing.

One thing is certain: the vertical buttons of the doctor's white coat have become the horizontal buttons on the left of the dentist's white coat, with a three- or four-button fastening. Polite and elegant, they require the complicity of the two hands in ancient, slow gestures which call for silence and atmosphere. They evoke the image of a doctor who, early in the morning, calmly buttons his white coat, gathering his thoughts in that professional gesture. A new way of wearing a smooth, optional-free white coat is being introduced: the garment is put on by being drawn over the head like a sweater, and it is slipped off in the same way, without buttons, pockets, stitching, or squiggles: it is the maximum of 'autoclavability' and of the minimum necessary.

The first 'mismatched outfits' began to appear in Italian dental practices in the early '80s in a new mix of fabrics, colours and accessories. The same is true for protective caps, packaged in the same colour as important protective devices. The 'dentist's' white coat has thus shaken off the collective unconscious that identified it as a work device in an essentially surgical role, as it was represented in eighteenth century painting.

Let us continue the inspectional and emotional analysis of the white coat. After having recalled the evolution of the dentist's white coat with respect to its closure mode, there came zippers–fast, modular, frontal.

Zippers, which also nowadays appear coloured, belong to the modern age, but at the same time to modern antiques, having received a big jolt from invasive Covid-19. Not recommended, being a potential viral receptacle, they seem destined to oblivion, like other objects formerly in vogue and now irremediably forgotten.

Example: does anyone remember suspenders? Are they still in use? Many objects have been retired by fashion trends. With the introduction of one-piece scrubs that can be put on over the head, we will certainly see the disappearance of zippers. But we will also see the disappearance of these slip-over scrubs, the latter being already banned in some European countries to avoid contamination of the face when changing.

Very easy to clean and perfectly autoclavable, if they become viable in the future with full-length disposable coveralls (still with strips for airtight closure), we will go back to slow, thoughtful manual buttoning.

If we interpret his thought well, also Michele Cassetta, valiant colleague of Almini, comes to similar conclusions. Dentist, as well as scientific journalist and former professor of "Medical-patient communication" at the Department of Medicine in Bologna, Cassetta looks beyond: "We do not know what will be in the future lab coats and uniforms- he writes- because the medicine of artificial intelligence will change forever the relationship between doctor and patient. But many believe that precisely because machines will do many things better than us, the moment of human relationship and the value of rites and symbols will become even more important."

Chapter 13

DEVICE OR NOT DEVICE?

Is the white coat a device? There are many health professionals–observes Maria Sofia Rini, Legal Dentist, Professor of Applied Hygiene at the University of Bologna–who believe it is a device to protect oneself from the risk of infection. But if the white coat 'insulates', she says, it does not have a specific antibacterial power nor are there any national or European reference standards or guidelines with indications and/or suggestions. International references are often not homogeneous and do not refer to shared standards.

OSHA (Occupational Safety and Health Administration) mandates long sleeves and collared scrubs in the US, while Germany mandates short sleeves, as does almost all of Europe (except Italy, Croatia and Greece). Northern Europe forbids surgical scrubs removable over the head, while Germany and northern countries have rules regarding washing, maintenance and/or choice of colour. These are all local and regional rules, however, whose scientific and regulatory validity is not shared.

If white, as everyone knows, identifies health professions as a symbol of cleanliness and hygiene, sterility is not required in outpatient clinics. The lack of unambiguous rules excludes that the classic white coat can fall within the context of the Medical Devices for Protection from Biological Risk regulated in Europe by the new European Regulation No. 425/2016-DPI or in PPE, Personal Protective Equipment class III, to which the role of protection from risk is recognised.

In the healthcare field, professional attire should ensure professionalism through health protection as per prior risk assessment. Regarding some surgical activities, including those of outpatient nature, it should meet suitability requirements and, on the basis of the risk assessment, be treated as a PPE (Personal Protective Equipment, L81/2008), then assimilated to equipment or devices to protect the health and safety of those who wear or use them (Legislative Decree 475/92).

EU Regulation No. 425/2016 includes white coats or uniforms among Category 1 PPE, i.e. among those that 'protect against minimal risks'. In the absence of particular risks or risks recognised as such, protection of the body (total and/or partial) is therefore entrusted to business attire/work clothing having such features as to provide a decent defense/insulation from a hygienic/protective point of view and from environmental stresses (of thermal, atmospheric and, powdery nature).

However, professional clothing for ordinary use must comply with certain basic safety and standardisation requirements defined by UNI-EN 340 in respect of ergonomics, resistance, and minimum number of sizes available. They must be EC marked in a visible and indelible manner, and the product must be accompanied by a statement of the manufacturer in Italian.

The Italian and European regulatory framework in general do not clearly identify the characteristics dictated by technical standards of reference. Therefore, ordinary sanitary professional attire in Italy CAN'T be considered a device even if it can be a good form of 'risk containment'.

One is the contraction of 'Occupational Infectious Diseases' by dentists and staff, because in dentistry, contact with the microbial population of the oral cavity, blood, and saliva is close. However, the proper choice, proper use and effective treatment/maintenance of professional clothing is an additional element of protection.

In stressing the importance of protection and prevention, the Consolidated Act on safety in the workplace (Law 81/2008, chapter II art. 74) seems to exclude sanitary clothing, defining PPE as 'any equipment designed to be worn by the worker to protect him/her against one or more risks likely to threaten safety or health during work, as well as any complement or accessory designed for that purpose.'

The standard provides clear guidance but is not sector specific. It is up to the employer and the competent doctor to identify potential risks when drawing up the assessment document. In essence, the standard leaves the issue open to the variability of situations and assessments which are to be motivated and documented.

Considering the new European Regulation (already implemented on MDs), the request for a category II or III certification for ordinary sanitary clothing seems impractical: there are too many obligations and certifications that would increase production and market costs by imposing too strict management rules.

In excluding sanitary professional clothing, the legislation has only considered gloves, protective eyewear, face masks etc. Law 81/2008 states that PPE (Article 76) 'must be made appropriate to the working conditions' and take into account the ergonomic or health needs of the worker; but since 1990 (Ministerial Decree of September 28, 1990 on 'Standards for protection from professional HIV infection in public and private health and welfare facilities') the obligation has only applied to gloves in use during dental procedures, without considering health uniforms.

Subsequently, DM 28/09/1990 and the 1994 circular of the Ministry of Health with the 'Practical recommendations for the control of infections in dentistry' addressed the infectious problem in a more systematic way, without changing anything substantially.

The most serious manufacturers provide data sheets on the characteristics and maintenance of the sanitary uniforms they market. According to the European Regulation, they indicate them as 'protective clothing for minor risks', i.e. 'professional uniforms for general use only for minimal risks, in particular in terms of ergonomics, non-harmfulness, comfort' (1ST. Category PPE with reference to Legislative Decree 475/92), excluding 'liability for the claim of protection from risks other than those contemplated in the specific information note.'

The identification and choice of a uniform best suited to the risk in the workplace shall be made by the employer and those who identify the type of risk, knowing that 'the garment does not protect against risks arising from burns, abrasions, mechanical aggression (e.g. cuts), chemical aggression (acids, solvents etc.), exposure to infectious agents and risks for which the PPE has not been certified'.

EU Regulation No. 425/2016 expands the requirements, the level of safety and the specifications to be met. It recognises the importance of healthcare clothing complying with pre-established technical features and rules (cat. I PPE), more cogent rules and checks in case of greater and specific risks (cat. III). But on what basis and in what terms will risk and protection be assessed in a context of healthcare activities that differ in their purpose and method of execution?

It must be admitted that professionals today do not seem to pay enough attention to this issue. They seem to be more concerned about costs than risk assessment choices, given that stricter regulation would lead to fears of unreasonable and not always justified increases. If the white coat is not a device, there are fears that the risk, especially in dentistry, may be underestimated to the advantage of marketing or image.

A solution could be the presence of disposable scrubs, sterile or not, on the market, although the safety required by such devices will weigh even on such a choice. In addition to appearing aesthetically unpleasant, they may not prove to be cheaper in the long run. If properly and appropriately used (single-patient), the disposable fabric/non-woven or synthetic would provide a good barrier effect, but to the detriment of breathability, wearability, and comfort.

Although medical clothing is not considered a device, it plays an important role in the profession and the management of specific professional risks. If on the one hand it does not justify high costs, on the other hand the purchase of medical uniforms, without specific certifications and information, is not allowed either.

Chapter 14

THE DIFFICULT CHOICE BETWEEN A MEDICAL DEVICE (MD) AND A PERSONAL PROTECTIVE EQUIPMENT (PPE)

Until the mid-'80s, there was no real specific legislation on occupational health and safety in Europe. A first important turning point occurred in 1987 with the drafting of the Single European Act, marked by the introduction of a new legal provision aimed at promoting 'improvements to protect the safety and health of workers'. Subsequently, with the Treaty of Amsterdam, in 1997, the provisions on the Occupational Safety and Health standards (OSHA) were defined within the TEU.

Before the pandemic, medical clothing was generally considered only a symbol or a mild protection, and few took the trouble to verify if white coats, visors, gloves, and caps were PPE (Personal Protective Equipment) or even MD (Medical Device) and were properly informed about the rules to which a doctor and his staff were subjected.

It is necessary to consider that medical offices, clinics, and hospitals represent a complex reality from a regulatory point of view. In fact, managers are obliged to provide PPE that guarantees the operator's protection and, at the same time, if the operator's function requires it, they must guarantee the patient's protection through the use of medical devices.

Unfortunately, in the field of medical clothing, PPE and MDs, due to their nature and the degree of protection they offer, are rarely bivalent and the health crisis has generated a series of rules, guidelines and various precautions which have inevitably increased personal fears of possibly unsuitable protective measures. The entire industry has found itself faced with the obligation to fully understand not only the legislative norms, but also the specific features of each PPE and MD in order to evaluate their relative efficacy.

Our poor white coat, to which this book is dedicated, has quickly gone from being an 'almost' article of clothing to a protective device or a medical device depending on its use and since 2020 it has been covered by overalls and scrubs in 'non-woven fabric' that had to perform the double protection and that have caused serious discomfort to operators as well as an image that has created considerable anxiety in patients.

Without entering into the distinction of what and how to use these protections, there is no doubt that from now on the concept of white coat will no longer be the same as in the past and we must prepare ourselves for a 'revolution' that will change the physician's image in a substantial way. It will oblige him to constantly check the technical features even of an article considered until yesterday of minor importance and assumed to be a real health protection shield.